THOUGHTS AND FEELINGS

How to Bring Your Thoughts and Feelings Back to the Present

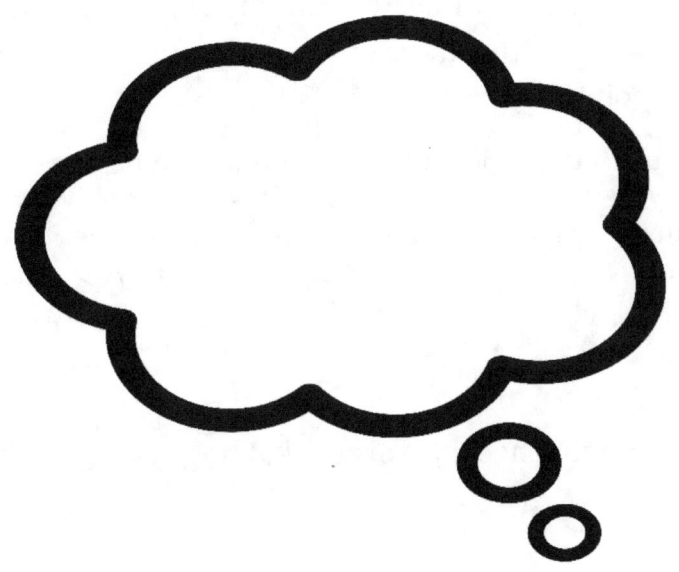

BY: Patricia A. Carlisle

Introduction

I want to thank you and congratulate you for choosing the book, "**THOUGHTS AND FEELINGS: *How to Bring Your Thoughts and Feelings back to the Present***".

This book contains proven steps and strategies on how to use the power of your mind to forget about pain and disappointment.

Everyone has things from the past that are hunting our present. Letting go and living in the moment is not as easy as it sounds. However, it is not an impossible mission. It's amazing how many thing we can change if we really want. Learn how to use the power of your mind to forget about pain and disappointment.

In order to change your mind set and let the past stay where it belongs, you need to do some exercises. Imagine your brain is like a muscle. If you want to improve and change it, you need to exercise it. Follow these easy steps to help you get over any traumas or painful events from the past.

Thanks again for choosing this book, I hope you enjoy it!

TABLE OF CONTENT

Chapter 1

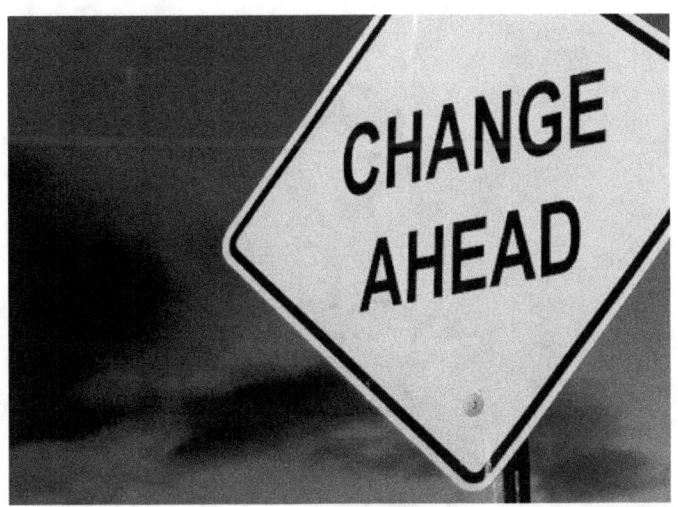

CHANGE YOUR MIND SET

As you probably know, happiness is a relative notion. As human beings, we can easily find reasons to complain and be unhappy. No matter how many successes you have, you will always look back at the things you didn't get in life. There is nothing wrong with looking back at the things you didn't get in life as long as you don't let it influence your present. The best you can do is to take the bad things from the past and let them fuel you with motivation in the future. However, instead of doing this you focus on how unlucky you are, there is nothing to gain.

In order to change your mind set and let the past stay where it belongs, you need to do some exercises. Imagine your brain is a muscle. If you want to improve and change it, you need to exercise it. Follow these easy steps to help you get over any traumas or painful events from the past.

Chapter 2

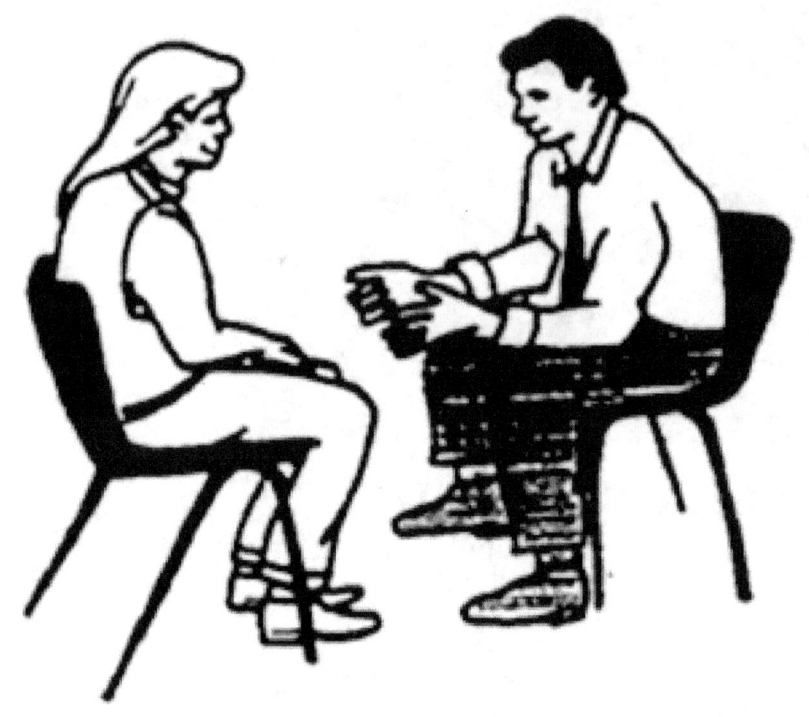

LET IT ALL OUT

If something that happened a while ago is still bothering you, the worst thing you can do is to keep it all in. You need to talk about it. If you have a partner, communicate your thoughts and feelings with him or her.

In case you are single, talk to your friends or family. If you make the first step, they might get the courage to share with you their pain and fears too. This will make you feel that you are not alone. You cannot compare your experience with other people, but it always helps to remember you are not the only one suffering. Others might be going through worst experiences and they are learning how to get over it. This should motivate and inspire you.

If you feel you cannot trust anyone or you don't want to burden your loved ones, you can always talk to a therapist. It is amazing how just talking about things that make you unhappy can free you. Communicate your negative feelings and you will feel how they transform into new positive energy.

You cannot keep things bottled up inside forever. At some point they will explode and the consequences might be huge.

The person listening doesn't even have to say anything. As soon as you share all your thoughts, you will have a feeling of intense relief. It will be like someone took a heavy stone off your chest.

If you are one of those people who find it hard to open up and talk to someone, do not worry. You can always pick up a pen and paper and just send an old fashioned letter to a friend or family member. You can have the face to face conversation after he or she read your letter and has all the facts. You can of course use your email for this too.

Chapter 3

Riches flow into my life

USE POSITIVE AFFIRMATIONS

Positive affirmations are more powerful than you think. This is like training your brain to believe what you are saying. At first, the affirmations might sound like empty words. After a while, you end up believing the words you say. To get over what happened to you in the past and be happy right now, you can say an affirmation like this:

"I am strong and happy. What happened in the past cannot affect me today. Right now I am the luckiest person alive. I am grateful for all the good things in my life."

Say this affirmation while looking at you in the mirror. Make eye contact with yourself and make sure you sound and look like you really mean what you are saying. At first it will feel like lying, but eventually you will end up believing your words. Do not expect to achieve this in a couple of days. It takes a lot of practice and motivation. Do your affirmations twice a day.

Start in the morning before breakfast. This will give you a boost of good energy for the rest of your day. And end your days with positive affirmations too.

Make a list with all the things you have good in your life. At first, if you are really sad, it might feel there is nothing good in the present. However, try to focus a little better. Think about all the people who love you. If you are healthy, do not take that for granted. If you take your time, you will find a long list with great things you should be grateful for. Repeat the list while you say your affirmations.

To understand better how this works, let's take an example. Imagine a woman who cannot have children no matter how much she wishes. In the past, she had a miscarriage and she cannot get over it. The woman is thinking about it every single day and this makes her unhappy in the present. However, she forgets about all the amazing things she already has in her life. She has a great man who loves her more than anything.

Except for infertility, she also has her health. The woman has a successful career and a lot of people who care for her. However, she is unable to enjoy any of these things until she lets go of the past. Her positive affirmation should include all these good things. She could also say to herself that she is strong enough to move past infertility and be happy right now.

Chapter 4

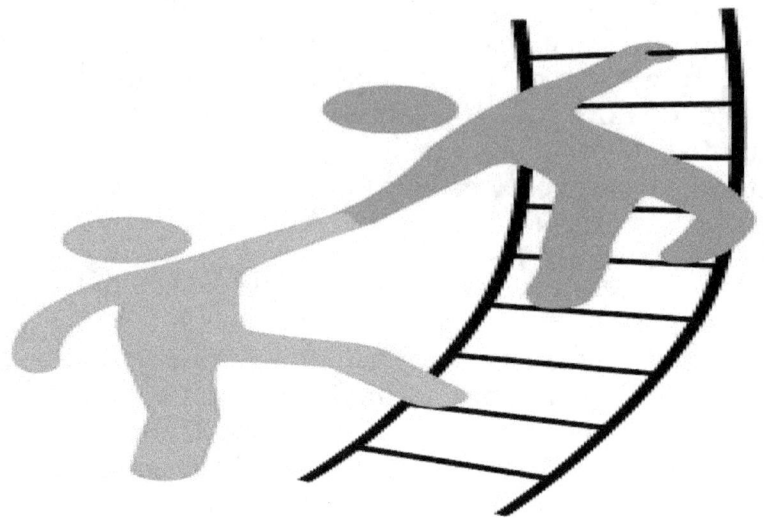

HELP OTHER PEOPLE

Spending so much time thinking about the past is not good for you. To get your mind off problems, one of the best solutions is to try to help other people. There is nothing more fulfilling than knowing that you helped someone. It's always easier to deal with other's problems any way. If someone needs help, spend all your energy trying to help them. This does not mean you need to fix everything that is wrong in the world. Sometimes people just need to know you are there for them.

After you help someone in need, your own issues become a lot smaller. It is also possible not to have any time left for obsessing over the past. You will be too busy trying to make someone happy. In the process you will end up making yourself happy too.

By getting involved in other person's life, you might discover that your own troubles are actually insignificant by comparison. Of course this will not please you but it will help you put things in perspective.

Get involved in charity cases. It's not enough just to donate money to feel better. You need to get involved and get to know those people. Learn their stories and get inspired. This does not mean your past is any less painful.

However, it will show you how other people manage to leave their problems behind. If you don't have the possibility to help with charity cases, you can just help a friend in need. If you know someone who is going through something difficult, pick up the phone and call them. You might make them feel better just by asking if they are doing okay. You're showing them that someone cares. This is exactly what you needed in the past too.

Chapter 5

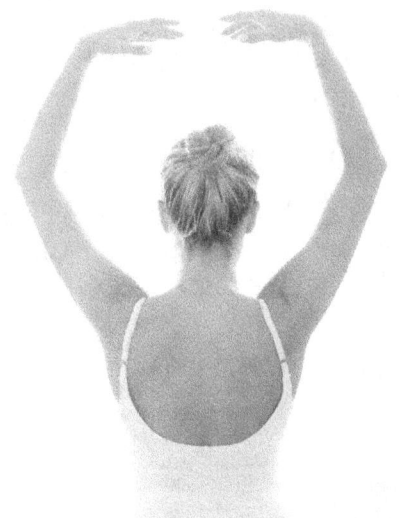

USE RELAXATION TECHNIQUES

Use relaxation techniques to move past the disappointments from yesterday and enjoy the happiness from today. These techniques will differ from everyone. It depends on what makes you relax. Think about what you like to do at the end of a long day. For example, if you enjoy watching a TV show, just take the day off, get some delicious snacks and watch your favorite show all day long. Music has the power to change your mood and relax you too.

Make yourself a nice warm bath and put some of your favorite music on. Escape from the reality for a few hours or even for a few minutes every day. Take time for yourself and recharge your batteries. Physical activity is also beneficial when it comes to relieving stress and leaving the past behind. Exercising help the body release a special type of hormone which creates a relaxing and happy feeling.

Nature is also very soothing and relaxing. Spend some time on the beach and just watch the waves. Go in the forest with your dog for a long walk. Another easy way to let go and have fun is by playing with children. If you have kids you should take your time and play with them. Children are almost always happy. Grownups lose this ability somewhere on a long the road. Learn from children how to be truly happy with the small things in life.

A night out with your friends, a weekend gateway with your loved one, or even a few extra hours of sleep can make a huge difference in your life. Just do whatever you want for once. Forget about work and other obligations. Take a few sick days if you feel depressed and stuck in the past. People often minimize the importance of psychological health. Sadness is a first step towards depression and this should be taken seriously.

Chapter 6

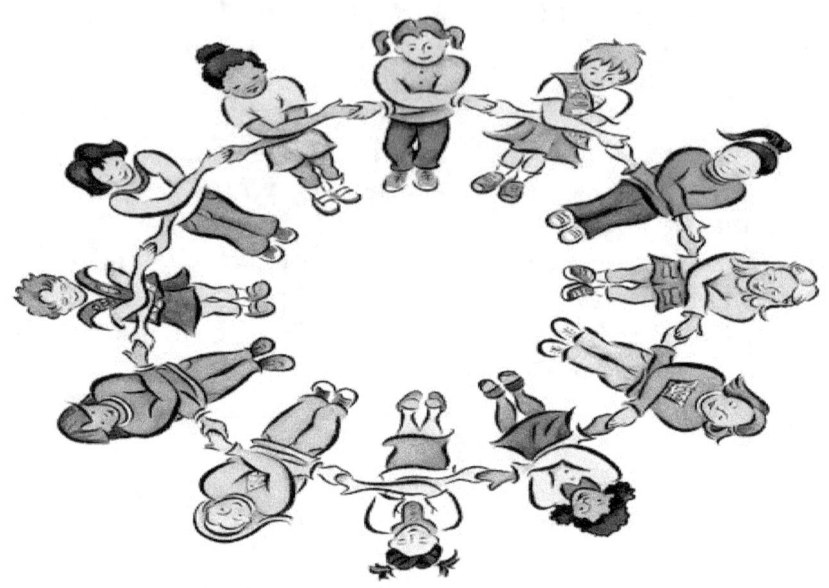

LOOK FOR OTHER PEOPLE WHO SHARE YOUR PAIN

There are a lot of other people in your situation. If you don't know them in your life, search online. Join chats or forums where you can get to know their stories and share your own experience. If you talk to someone who's been through the same traumatic experience like you did, you might find the comfort you need to move on.

Sometimes it can be difficult to talk to someone who has never been through the same things. They can be sympathetic but they can never really understand. People need to feel understood in order to get over something painful. Another reason to find someone who knows what you been through is to get motivated. You will see that other people were able to find the strength to move on and you might discover some good tips.

By using the internet to chat with people, you will feel safe. Nobody knows who you are and nobody can see you. It's just you and your computer. On the other side is another person who knows exactly how you feel. This can be even more freeing than talking to someone face to face. Most people can express their feelings and inner thoughts a lot easier in writing. Even if you get no tips on how to move past it, just knowing that another person went through the exact same thing will make you feel ten times better. You will feel less alone.

Chapter 7

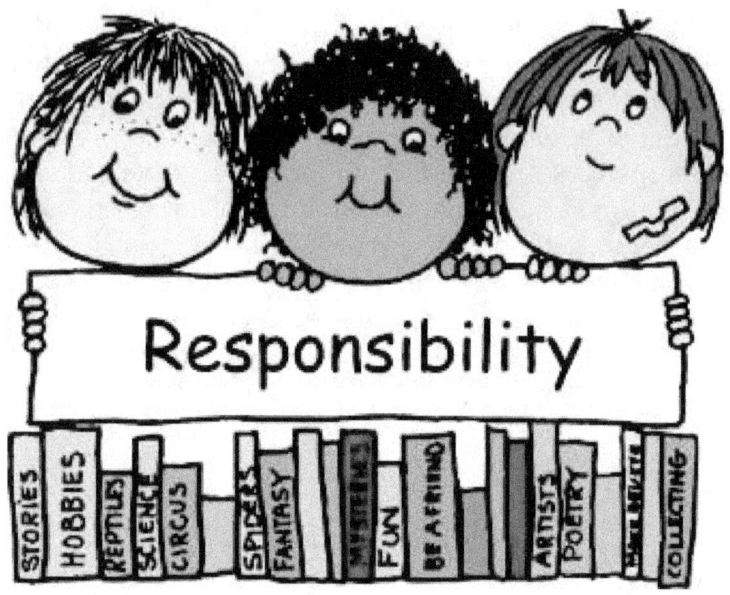

ACCEPT YOUR RESPONSIBILITY FOR THE PAST

In order to move past something you need to accept responsibility for your part of guilt. You cannot blame everyone else. You shouldn't blame yourself either. You should just take a long look at yourself and see if there is something you need to take responsibility for. Once you know what you did wrong you can use that experience to learn from your mistake. This is what the saying, half full of the glass means. You take a negative situation and you use it to create something good.

Let's imagine the painful event from your past has something to do with a fight you had with someone you love. Even if that person has most of the blame, you need to search carefully and see if there is something you did wrong too. You're only human and it's impossible to do everything right.

Taking responsibility for your actions in this case means going to that person and apologizing. This will make you feel so much better. It does't even matter if that person will not apologies too. You are doing this for yourself. It is your way of taking responsibility and moving toward a brighter future. Do not be too proud to do this. It is understandable that saying "I am sorry" is not an easy thing to do. Actually, most people find it very difficult. If you manage to get past this, you will feel much better. You will actually feel lighter, as if you left an ugly part of you behind.

Chapter 8

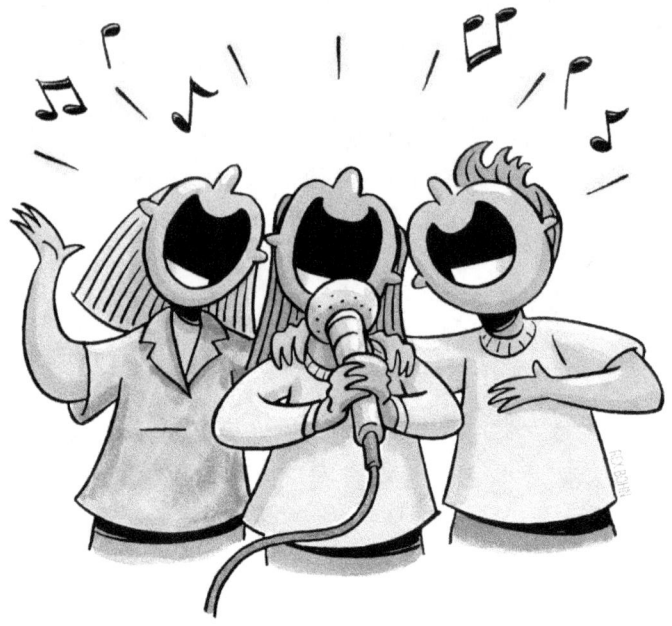

LIVE IN THE MOMENT

Living in the moment sounds a lot easier said than done. You can achieve this only if you really try. This means that you

have to put all your focus on what is happening today. Don't think about the past or the future. All that matters is now. Are you now having fun with your children and family? Be happy for this. Tomorrow is another day and you need to take things day by day.

You can also use work as a distraction from sad memories. Instead of dwelling on what happened some time ago, focus to make your career a success. The satisfaction you will get from this will make you feel good about yourself. Working is a type of therapy too. If you don't have a job, you can use house work for this. You can clean the house or cook for your loved ones. Organize a big family dinner with all your relatives. If you have a big family, this will keep you busy enough and will leave you absolutely no time for thinking of the past. Making your family happy with a reunion and a delicious dinner will give you a lot of joy too.

Another way to keep your mind in the present is getting involved in a project you enjoy. This can be anything. For example you can organize a party with the neighbors, you can get involved in school projects with your friends or you can help out your local church.

Chapter 9

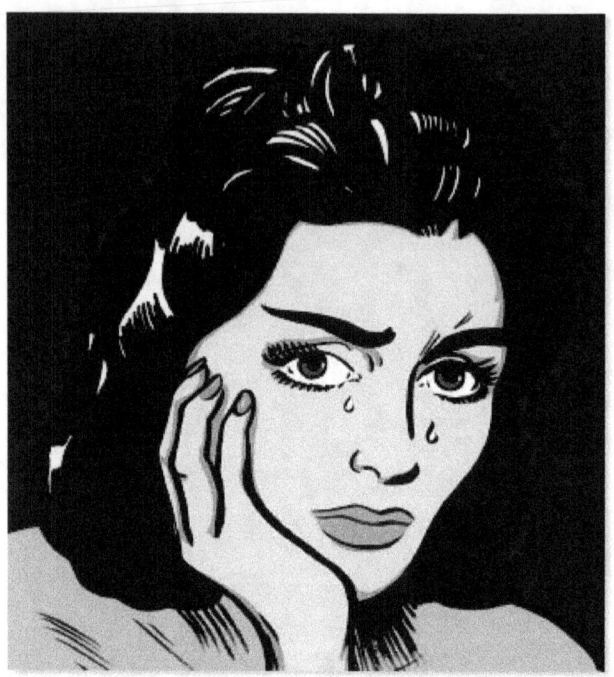

DO NOT PITY YOURSELF

By pitying yourself and saying "poor me", you will only succeed to feel worse. There are times in life when you need to be hard on yourself. For example, if you feel too depressed to see anyone, do it way. Being surrounded by people always helps. Do not stay alone with your bad memories and dark thoughts. Try to find some company. If you are home alone, go visit some friends. Even talking on the phone with someone helps if there is no way to meet them that day.

Watching something fun on TV instead of recycling old memories is also something you should consider. Do anything that give your pleasure and helps you focus on the present. If you feel you are too deep in sadness and you don't have the power to get rid of it, ask for professional help. There is absolutely no shame in this. This would not mean that you pity yourself. It would mean that you admit you have a problem and you have the courage to ask for help and do something about it. With most problems, the first step is recognizing and admitting. If you are in denial you risk falling in a depression

Chapter 10

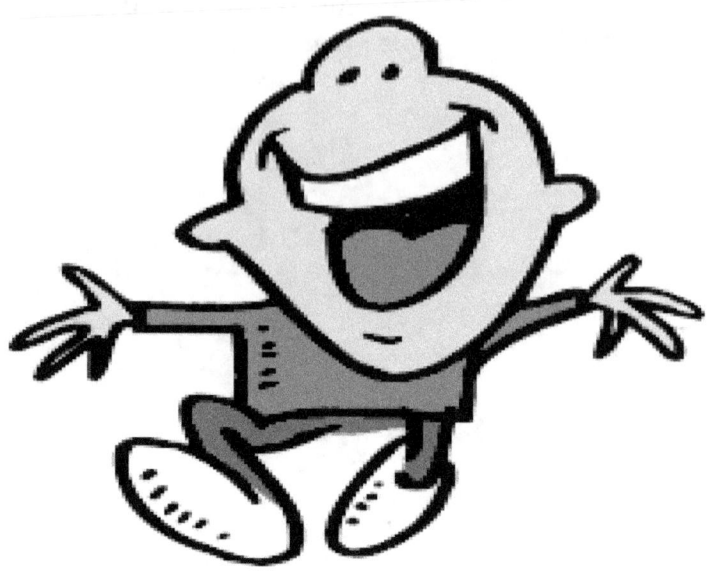

FUN THERAPY

Do something fun with your family and try to laugh more. There is no better therapy than laughing. To avoid sad memories, try to stay away from triggers. For example, you can avoid places that remind you of that specific bad thing. You should also stay away from sad movies. Get some comedies you know would make you laugh. Watch them with your friends. Another way to have fun is of course by throwing a party. Just dance and have a blast for a few hours. This is the best method to help you live in the moment and be happy. Remember that happiness can last even for just a moment. It is up to you to make your days filled with happy moments.

Make a list with all the things you love to do. Having fun is different for everyone. This is why you should make your own personalized list. Having that list somewhere where you can see it every day and try to do at least one thing. Keep in mind that you are the only one who can make you happy. Other people can help too but you should never depend on anyone.

If you put all your hopes and dreams on one person you might get disappointed. Why should you give that kind of power over you to anyone? Take control over your life and enjoy it.

Chapter 11

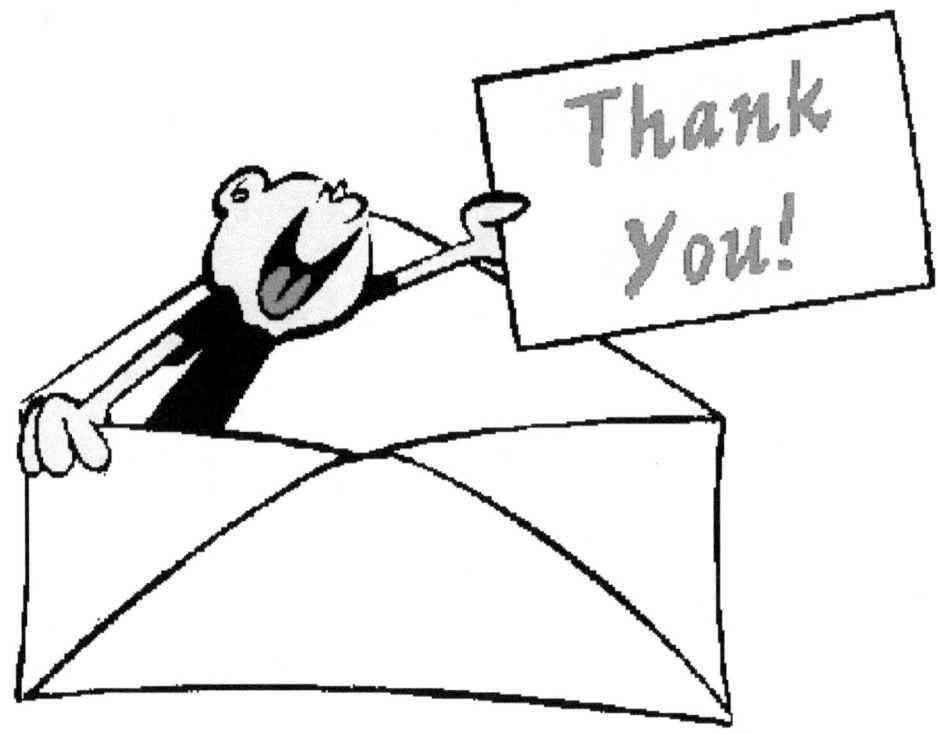

SAY THANK YOU

If you look back you will see that you are not alone. You have people in your life who have always been there. Instead of crying about what happened, take some time to be grateful and thank them for all their support. Without them maybe your day would be much worse.

By thanking them, you remind yourself that you are loved. Knowing this, will give you the force you need to get up, dust yourself off and move on with your life.

Conclusion

Thank you again for choosing this book!

I hope this book was able to help you learn how to live and enjoy life with intensity.

By remembering the painful past over and over again, you are relieving it. It's like going through that bad situation every single day. Why would you want this? Embrace your past and be grateful for what you have in the present. This is what living and enjoying life with intensity means.

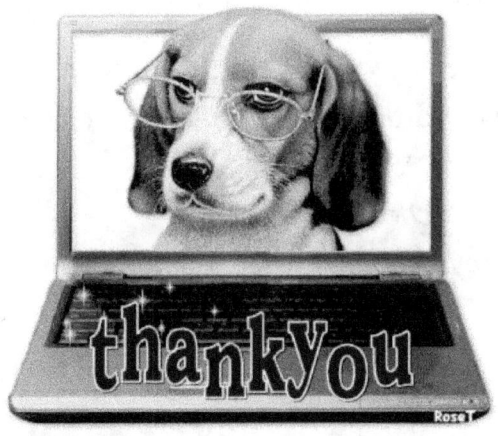

Finally, if you enjoyed this book, would you be kind enough to leave a review for this book on Amazon? It'd be greatly appreciated!

Thank you and good luck!

Preview Of 'Positive Affirmations for a Better Life: Let the magic begin!'

POSITIVE AFFIRMATIONS

When you feel lonely and sad:

1. I feel the love of those who are not physically around me.

2. I take pleasure in my own solitude.

3. I am too big a gift to this world to feel self-pity.

4. I love and approve of myself.

When you feel terrified (without your safety being in danger):

5. I focus on breathing and grounding myself.

6. Following my intuition and my heart keeps me safe and sound.

7. I make the right choices every time.

8. I draw from my inner strength and light.

9. I trust myself.

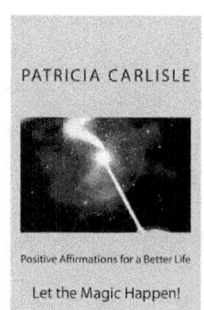

POSITIVE AFFIRMATIONS FOR A BETTER LIFE. LET THE MAGIC HAPPEN!

Check Out My Other Books

Below you'll find some of my other popular books that are popular on Amazon and Kindle as well. Alternatively, you can visit my author page on Amazon to see other work done by me.

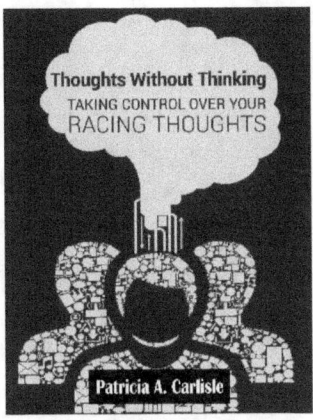

Thoughts Without Thinking: Taking control over your racing thoughts.

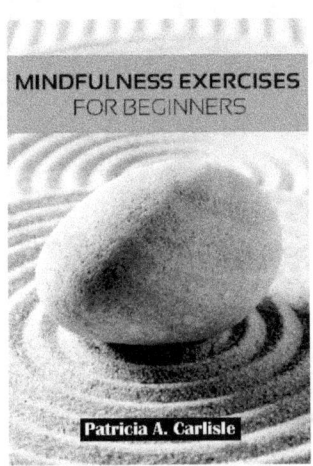

Mindfulness Exercises For Beginners (mindfulness, mindfulness for beginners.

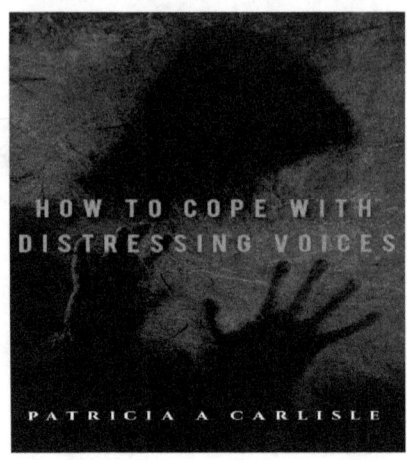

HOW TO COPE WITH DISTRESSING VOICES.

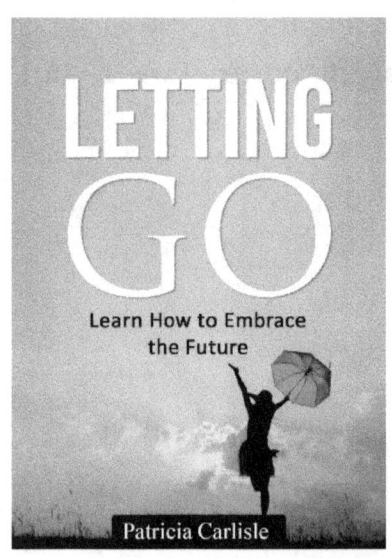

LETTING GO: LEARN HOW TO EMBRACE THE FUTURE.

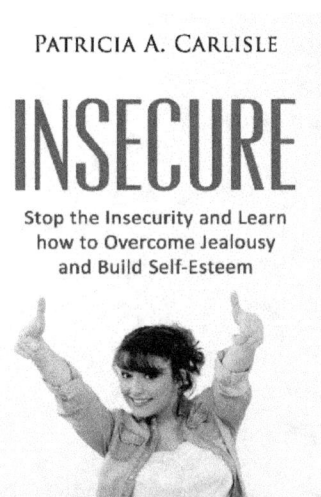

INSECURE: STOP THE INSECURITY AND LEARN HOW TO OVERCOME JEALOUSY AND BUILD SELF-ESTEEM.

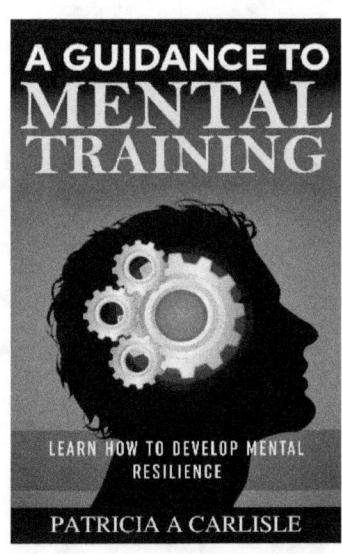

A GUIDANCE TO MENTAL TRAINING: LEARN HOW TO DEVELOP MENTAL RESILIENCE.

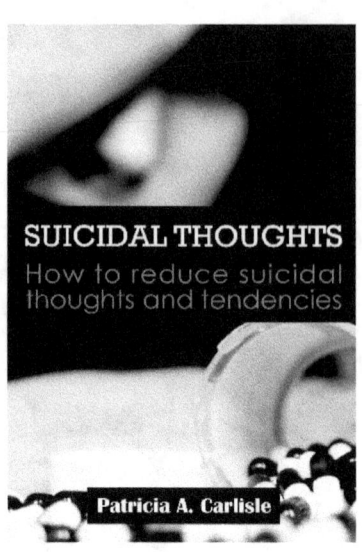

SUICIDAL THOUGHTS: HOW TO REDUCE SUICIDAL THOUGHTS AND TENDENCIES.

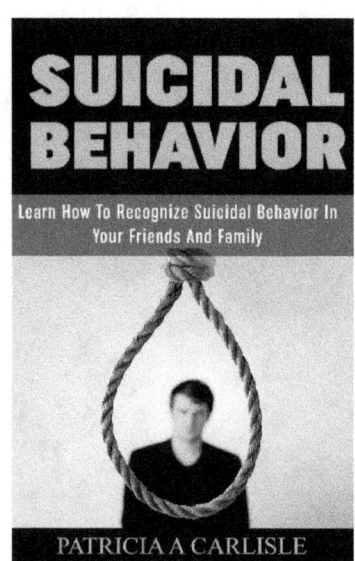

SUICIDAL BEHAVIOR: LEARN HOW TO RECOGNIZE SUICIDAL BEHAVIOR IN YOUR FRIENDS AND FAMILY.

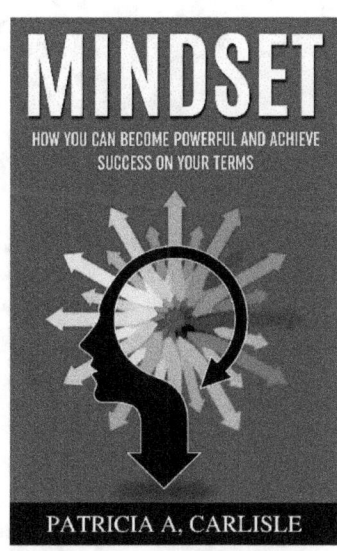

MINDSET: HOW YOU CAN BECOME POWERFUL AND ACHIEVE SUCCESS ON YOUR TERMS.

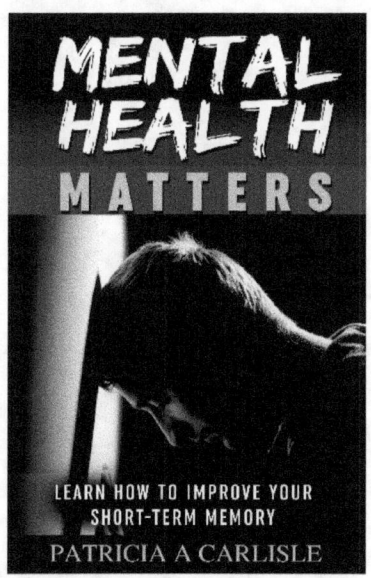

MENTAL HEALTH MATTERS: LEARN HOW TO IMPROVE YOUR SHORT-TERM MEMORY.

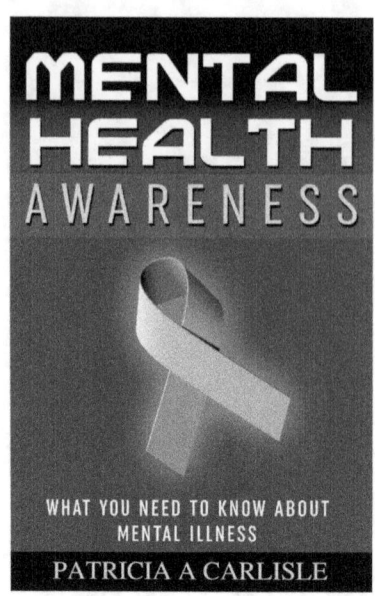

MENTAL HEALTH AWARENESS: WHAT YOU NEED TO KNOW ABOUT MENTAL ILLNESS.

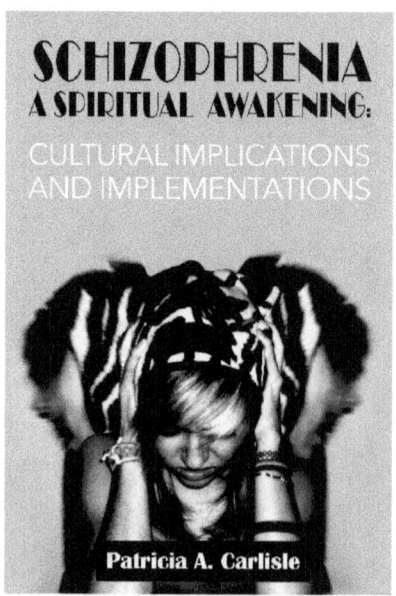

SCHIZOPHRENIA A SPIRITUAL AWAKENING: CULTURAL IMPLICATIONS AND IMPLEMENTATIONS.

BONUS: SUBSCRIBE TO THE FREE BOOK

Beginners Guide to Yoga & Meditation

"Stressed out? Do You Feel Like The World Is Crashing Down Around You? Want To Take A Vacation That Will Relax Your Mind, Body And Spirit? Well this Easy To Read Step By Step

E-Book Makes It All Possible!"

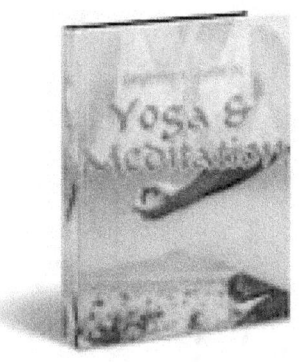

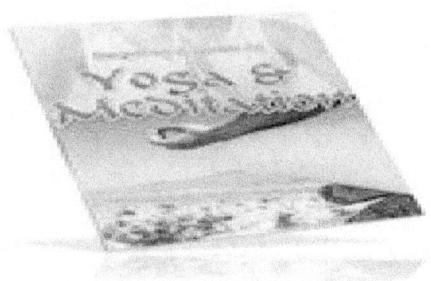

Instructions on how to join our mailing list, and receive a free copy of "Yoga and Meditation" can be found in any of my Kindle eBooks.

NOTES

NOTES

NOTES

NOTES

NOTES

www.ingramcontent.com/pod-product-compliance
Lightning Source LLC
Chambersburg PA
CBHW060344290526
45791CB00004B/1525